WHERE THERE IS NO VISION FROM GOD, THE PEOPLE RUN WILD, BUT THOSE WHO ADHERE TO GOD'S INSTRUCTION KNOW GENUINE HAPPINESS.

PROVERBS 29:18, THE VOICE

This wellness journal is for the person who believes that with God anything is possible but recognizes the need for intentionality. Living with a vision for each day fends off haste that makes waste and confusion that complicates things. A person who feels like they are getting nowhere lives frustrated, easily stumbles, and is most likely to give up on their hopes and dreams.

God has a vision and a plan for your life. It's a good and hopeful plan for the future.

"For I know the plans I have for you," declares the Lord, "plans to prosper you and not to harm you, plans to give you a hope and a future." – Jeremiah 29:11

The vision God gives for your life is bigger than anything you can ask or imagine. It begins in the day to day, the little by little. If you feel like you lack grand purposes or plans because you've been so darn busy trying to make it through another day, it's okay. This journal is for you. As you practice using this journal, little by little, you will hear God speak to you through His Word each day. In God's kingdom, little things hold tremendous power.

"Do not despise these small beginnings, for the LORD rejoices to see the work begin, to see the plumb line in Zerubbabel's hand." – Zechariah 4:10

The things God wants to do through you and for you don't come from working harder and checking off more boxes on your to-do list. Visions of a hopeful future come to pass as you allow Him to work through you with His empowering grace. This grace-empowered change requires your whole self – heart, mind, soul, and body. When we do as he commands, we partner with God to do good and hopeful things in the world.

"And you shall love the Lord your God with all your heart and with all your soul and with all your mind and with all your strength." – Mark 12:30

Every day, you have the opportunity to partner with God to bring hope to the world by providing a vision for the future. It's important to have a personal vision for each day.

Whether God is calling you to tend to your physical health, go back to school to get that degree, write the book, or do that scary thing, this journal is here to help.

All the goodness God gives starts with faith – a belief in what can't be seen yet. Some things God wants for us can't be seen right now. But with patience and daily tending to our mustard seed of faith, the watering of God's Word, followed up by action, visions come to pass. The key is to stay faithful to the process of faith. The unseen will become seen.

This journal is here to help you be well; to stay faithful to God's Word and the process of faith.

HOW TO USE THIS JOURNAL

Each day you will:

WRITE THE WORD: Begin with writing down the Word. You can always use the YouVersion app or any daily Bible verse app to find your verse. If you're already going through a Bible reading plan or particular Bible study, pick a verse that pops out and grabs your attention. If you're not involved in an organized study plan, simply open your Bible and read God's Word until a verse grabs your attention. This attention-grabbing moment is the Holy Spirit in action, highlighting something God wants you to know.

SOAK IN THE WORD: Take 2-3 minutes to settle down, sit, and breathe. Set a timer on your phone if needed. Inhale and exhale as you meditate on the Word. Fill your mind with the Word of God. This is called "soaking." Soaking is not to be confused with studying God's Word. Soaking in God's Word is like receiving a warm hug or kind and loving correction. Remember, His words are never ones of shame or fear. Take this time to let your imagination run with God. He wants to speak and show you good things.

WRING IT OUT: Once you've soaked, like a sponge in fresh, cool water, now it's time to wring it out. Write down how this particular piece of scripture applies to your day.

TODAY I AM GRATEFUL FOR: List three things you are grateful for. Gratitude has been proven to upgrade our immune systems and improve our brain-body connection so we can act, feel, and think as whole and integrated people - people of peace. Gratitude requires you to take account of what God has done so you can operate from contentment: a restful state of being rather than a selfish, close-fisted, striving, and fearful state. Gratitude reminds your soul that you are a child of God, an heir of God and co-heir of Christ, and keeps your pride from showing up with something to prove throughout the day.

TOP THREE THINGS TO DO TODAY: Write down three things to do each day– things that get you closer to your vision. Perhaps start with things you have been procrastinating and putting off. A recent study showed that people who write things down are 42% more likely to complete the task. As children of God, we don't accomplish things to prove ourselves good to God, yet God gives every person a specific gift and a calling. God wants to see you fulfill the call and vision He has for your life. Work never produces faith, but faith naturally produces work. List your top three things for each day, then come back and check them off when you complete them!

WHAT I NEED FOR MY MIND: Ask the Holy Spirit what kind of thoughts you need for the day and what you will think when something comes against your vision.

WHAT I NEED FOR MY EMOTIONS: Ask the Holy Spirit what kind of feelings you need and what to do when feelings show up and don't support the vision for the day.

WHAT I NEED FOR MY SOUL: Your soul makes you, YOU! It holds your unique will and desires in light of the life experiences you have had. Biblically it's known as the seat of your thoughts, will, and emotions. Our souls need direction. Tell it how to go and do God's vision for your life. Write down what your soul needs to keep you dreaming and desiring big!

WHAT I NEED FOR MY BODY: Our bodies give us the ability to do what needs to get done to carry out the vision for our lives. Our physical bodies make the unseen things of the spiritual realm seen. Our bodies need energy (aka..input, fuel, liquids, food) to do work. What kind of fuel does your body need to do what you desire to get done?

MOVEMENT: Neuroscience confirms that our bodies and brains are connected. When our bodies move, our brains have a chance to create NEW neuropathway grooves. Think of neuropathways as the habits of your brain – some good, some bad. To move towards the vision God has for our lives, we must stop some of these bad habits of our brain. We do this by starting new, healthy habits for our minds. Movement is like medicine for the thoughts we have that cause us pain and create bad habits in our brain. Daily movement doesn't have to be an intense, full-bore workout to create change. All movement counts. Each day, be thoughtful and intentional about how you will use movement as medicine for your brain-body connection. We highly encourage you to use the Revelation Wellness podcast episodes known as REVING the Word for renewing your mind during movement.

WATER: Our bodies are 60% water. Our brains are 73% water. If your body is dehydrated, your brain will be too. A dehydrated body feels achy, and a dehydrated mind feels foggy. God designed our bodies to need water more than any other substance on the earth – even more than food. The vision and hope for your day are supported well through the simple act of drinking enough water. Make it your goal to drink ½ your body weight in ounces of water. Then come back and circle how much you had at the end of each day.

SLEEP: A good day starts the night before. Everything we do well begins from rest. Good rest. The average person needs eight hours of sound sleep per night. Some people feel great with seven, and some need closer to nine. Record the length and quality of sleep from the night before, then make the adjustments to your sleep schedule and routine as needed.

NOTES & REFLECTION: Use this space as you wish to reflect on the day.

⟫ DATE: ....

☐ **WRITE THE WORD:**

....

....

....

....

....

☐ **SOAK IN THE WORD:**
SIT. INHALE. EXHALE. MEDITATE ON THIS VERSE FOR 2-3 MINUTES.

☐ **WRING IT OUT:**
HOW CAN I APPLY THIS VERSE TODAY?

....

....

TODAY I AM GRATEFUL FOR:

1
....

....

2
....

....

3
....

....

TOP 3 THINGS TO DO TODAY:
AS YOU WRITE, VISUALIZE YOURSELF DOING THEM AND THE OUTCOME YOU HOPE FOR.

1
....

2
....

3
....

WHAT I NEED FOR MY MIND (THOUGHTS):

....
....
....

WHAT I NEED FOR MY EMOTIONS (FEELINGS):

....
....
....

WHAT I NEED FOR MY SOUL (DESIRES/DREAMS):

....
....
....

WHAT I NEED FOR MY BODY:

....
....
....

MOVEMENT:

....
....
....

WATER:
GOAL: 1/2 YOUR BODYWEIGHT IN OUNCES

SLEEP:
QUALITY: ☆ ☆ ☆ ☆ ☆ HOURS:.........

NOTES AND REFLECTIONS: «

....
....
....
....
....
....
....
....
....
....
....
....
....
....
....
....
....
....
....
....
....
....
....
....
....
....
....

⟫ DATE: ....

☐ WRITE THE WORD:

....
....
....
....
....

☐ SOAK IN THE WORD:
SIT. INHALE. EXHALE. MEDITATE ON THIS VERSE FOR 2-3 MINUTES.

☐ WRING IT OUT:
HOW CAN I APPLY THIS VERSE TODAY?

....
....

TODAY I AM GRATEFUL FOR:

1
....
....

2
....
....

3
....
....

TOP 3 THINGS TO DO TODAY:
AS YOU WRITE, VISUALIZE YOURSELF DOING THEM AND THE OUTCOME YOU HOPE FOR.

1
....
2
....
3
....

WHAT I NEED FOR MY MIND (THOUGHTS):

....

....

....

WHAT I NEED FOR MY EMOTIONS (FEELINGS):

....

....

....

WHAT I NEED FOR MY SOUL (DESIRES/DREAMS):

....

....

....

WHAT I NEED FOR MY BODY:

....

....

....

MOVEMENT:

....

....

....

WATER:
GOAL: 1/2 YOUR BODYWEIGHT IN OUNCES

SLEEP:
QUALITY: ☆ ☆ ☆ ☆ ☆ HOURS:.........

NOTES AND REFLECTIONS:

....

....

....

....

....

....

....

....

....

....

....

....

....

....

....

....

....

....

....

....

....

....

....

....

....

....

....

>> DATE: ....

☐ **WRITE THE WORD:**

....

....

....

....

....

☐ **SOAK IN THE WORD:**

SIT. INHALE. EXHALE. MEDITATE ON THIS VERSE FOR 2-3 MINUTES.

☐ **WRING IT OUT:**

HOW CAN I APPLY THIS VERSE TODAY?

....

....

TODAY I AM GRATEFUL FOR:

1 ....

....

2 ....

....

3 ....

....

TOP 3 THINGS TO DO TODAY:

AS YOU WRITE, VISUALIZE YOURSELF DOING THEM AND THE OUTCOME YOU HOPE FOR.

1 ....

2 ....

3 ....

WHAT I NEED FOR MY MIND (THOUGHTS):

....

....

....

WHAT I NEED FOR MY EMOTIONS (FEELINGS):

....

....

....

WHAT I NEED FOR MY SOUL (DESIRES/DREAMS):

....

....

....

WHAT I NEED FOR MY BODY:

....

....

....

MOVEMENT:

....

....

....

WATER:
GOAL: 1/2 YOUR BODYWEIGHT IN OUNCES

SLEEP:
QUALITY: ☆ ☆ ☆ ☆ ☆ HOURS: ....

NOTES AND REFLECTIONS:

....

....

....

....

....

....

....

....

....

....

....

....

....

....

....

....

....

....

....

....

....

....

....

....

....

....

》》 DATE: ....

☐ WRITE THE WORD:

....
....
....
....
....

☐ SOAK IN THE WORD:
SIT. INHALE. EXHALE. MEDITATE ON THIS VERSE FOR 2-3 MINUTES.

☐ WRING IT OUT:
HOW CAN I APPLY THIS VERSE TODAY?

....
....

TODAY I AM GRATEFUL FOR:

1
....
....

2
....
....

3
....
....

TOP 3 THINGS TO DO TODAY:
AS YOU WRITE, VISUALIZE YOURSELF DOING THEM AND THE OUTCOME YOU HOPE FOR.

1
....

2
....

3
....

WHAT I NEED FOR MY MIND (THOUGHTS):

....

....

....

WHAT I NEED FOR MY EMOTIONS (FEELINGS):

....

....

....

WHAT I NEED FOR MY SOUL (DESIRES/DREAMS):

....

....

....

WHAT I NEED FOR MY BODY:

....

....

....

MOVEMENT:

....

....

....

WATER:
GOAL: 1/2 YOUR BODYWEIGHT IN OUNCES

SLEEP:
QUALITY: ☆ ☆ ☆ ☆ ☆ HOURS:.........

NOTES AND REFLECTIONS: 《《

....

....

....

....

....

....

....

....

....

....

....

....

....

....

....

....

....

....

....

....

....

....

....

....

....

....

....

....

....

....

≫ DATE: ....

☐ **WRITE THE WORD:**

....

....

....

....

....

☐ **SOAK IN THE WORD:**
   SIT. INHALE. EXHALE. MEDITATE ON THIS VERSE FOR 2-3 MINUTES.

☐ **WRING IT OUT:**
   HOW CAN I APPLY THIS VERSE TODAY?

....

....

TODAY I AM GRATEFUL FOR:

| 1 |
....

| 2 |
....

| 3 |
....

TOP 3 THINGS TO DO TODAY:
AS YOU WRITE, VISUALIZE YOURSELF DOING THEM AND THE OUTCOME YOU HOPE FOR.

| 1 |
| 2 |
| 3 |

WHAT I NEED FOR MY MIND (THOUGHTS):

....

....

....

WHAT I NEED FOR MY EMOTIONS (FEELINGS):

....

....

....

WHAT I NEED FOR MY SOUL (DESIRES/DREAMS):

....

....

....

WHAT I NEED FOR MY BODY:

....

....

....

MOVEMENT:

....

....

....

WATER:
GOAL: 1/2 YOUR BODYWEIGHT IN OUNCES

SLEEP:
QUALITY: ☆ ☆ ☆ ☆ ☆ HOURS:..........

NOTES AND REFLECTIONS:

....

....

....

....

....

....

....

....

....

....

....

....

....

....

....

....

....

....

....

....

....

....

....

....

....

....

....

....

⟫ DATE: ....

☐ WRITE THE WORD:

....
....
....
....
....

☐ SOAK IN THE WORD:
SIT. INHALE. EXHALE. MEDITATE ON THIS VERSE FOR 2-3 MINUTES.

☐ WRING IT OUT:
HOW CAN I APPLY THIS VERSE TODAY?

....
....

TODAY I AM GRATEFUL FOR:

1
....

2
....

3
....

....

TOP 3 THINGS TO DO TODAY:
AS YOU WRITE, VISUALIZE YOURSELF DOING THEM AND THE OUTCOME YOU HOPE FOR.

1
....

2
....

3
....

WHAT I NEED FOR MY MIND (THOUGHTS):

....
....
....

WHAT I NEED FOR MY EMOTIONS (FEELINGS):

....
....
....

WHAT I NEED FOR MY SOUL (DESIRES/DREAMS):

....
....
....

WHAT I NEED FOR MY BODY:

....
....
....

MOVEMENT:

....
....
....

WATER:
GOAL: 1/2 YOUR BODYWEIGHT IN OUNCES

SLEEP:
QUALITY: ☆ ☆ ☆ ☆ ☆ HOURS:.........

NOTES AND REFLECTIONS: 《《

....
....
....
....
....
....
....
....
....
....
....
....
....
....
....
....
....
....
....
....
....
....
....
....

≫ DATE: ....

☐ WRITE THE WORD:

....

....

....

....

....

☐ SOAK IN THE WORD:

SIT. INHALE. EXHALE. MEDITATE ON THIS VERSE FOR 2-3 MINUTES.

☐ WRING IT OUT:

HOW CAN I APPLY THIS VERSE TODAY?

....

....

TODAY I AM GRATEFUL FOR:

1 ....

....

2 ....

....

3 ....

....

TOP 3 THINGS TO DO TODAY:

AS YOU WRITE, VISUALIZE YOURSELF DOING THEM AND THE OUTCOME YOU HOPE FOR.

1 ....

2 ....

3 ....

WHAT I NEED FOR MY MIND (THOUGHTS):

....
....
....

WHAT I NEED FOR MY EMOTIONS (FEELINGS):

....
....
....

WHAT I NEED FOR MY SOUL (DESIRES/DREAMS):

....
....
....

WHAT I NEED FOR MY BODY:

....
....
....

MOVEMENT:

....
....
....

WATER:

GOAL: 1/2 YOUR BODYWEIGHT IN OUNCES

SLEEP:
QUALITY: ☆ ☆ ☆ ☆ ☆ HOURS:..........

NOTES AND REFLECTIONS: ⟪

....
....
....
....
....
....
....
....
....
....
....
....
....
....
....
....
....
....
....
....
....
....
....
....
....
....
....

≫ DATE: ....

☐ WRITE THE WORD:

....
....
....
....
....

☐ SOAK IN THE WORD:
SIT. INHALE. EXHALE. MEDITATE ON THIS VERSE FOR 2-3 MINUTES.

☐ WRING IT OUT:
HOW CAN I APPLY THIS VERSE TODAY?

....
....

TODAY I AM GRATEFUL FOR:

1
....

2
....

3
....

TOP 3 THINGS TO DO TODAY:
AS YOU WRITE, VISUALIZE YOURSELF DOING THEM AND THE OUTCOME YOU HOPE FOR.

1
2
3

WHAT I NEED FOR MY MIND (THOUGHTS):

....

....

....

WHAT I NEED FOR MY EMOTIONS (FEELINGS):

....

....

....

WHAT I NEED FOR MY SOUL (DESIRES/DREAMS):

....

....

....

WHAT I NEED FOR MY BODY:

....

....

....

MOVEMENT:

....

....

....

WATER:
GOAL: 1/2 YOUR BODYWEIGHT IN OUNCES

SLEEP:
QUALITY: ☆ ☆ ☆ ☆ ☆ HOURS:.........

NOTES AND REFLECTIONS: ⟪

....

....

....

....

....

....

....

....

....

....

....

....

....

....

....

....

....

....

....

....

....

....

....

....

....

....

....

≫≫ DATE: ....

☐ WRITE THE WORD:

....

....

....

....

....

☐ SOAK IN THE WORD:
SIT. INHALE. EXHALE. MEDITATE ON THIS VERSE FOR 2-3 MINUTES.

☐ WRING IT OUT:
HOW CAN I APPLY THIS VERSE TODAY?

....

....

TODAY I AM GRATEFUL FOR:

1
....

2
....

3
....

TOP 3 THINGS TO DO TODAY:
AS YOU WRITE, VISUALIZE YOURSELF DOING THEM AND THE OUTCOME YOU HOPE FOR.

1
2
3

WHAT I NEED FOR MY MIND (THOUGHTS):

....

....

....

WHAT I NEED FOR MY EMOTIONS (FEELINGS):

....

....

....

WHAT I NEED FOR MY SOUL (DESIRES/DREAMS):

....

....

....

WHAT I NEED FOR MY BODY:

....

....

....

MOVEMENT:

....

....

....

WATER:
GOAL: 1/2 YOUR BODYWEIGHT IN OUNCES

SLEEP:
QUALITY: ☆ ☆ ☆ ☆ ☆ HOURS:.........

NOTES AND REFLECTIONS: ≪

....

....

....

....

....

....

....

....

....

....

....

....

....

....

....

....

....

....

....

....

....

....

....

....

≫ DATE: ....

☐ WRITE THE WORD:

....
....
....
....
....

☐ SOAK IN THE WORD:
SIT. INHALE. EXHALE. MEDITATE ON THIS VERSE FOR 2-3 MINUTES.

☐ WRING IT OUT:
HOW CAN I APPLY THIS VERSE TODAY?

....
....

TODAY I AM GRATEFUL FOR:

1
....
....

2
....
....

3
....
....

TOP 3 THINGS TO DO TODAY:
AS YOU WRITE, VISUALIZE YOURSELF DOING THEM AND THE OUTCOME YOU HOPE FOR.

1
....
2
....
3
....

WHAT I NEED FOR MY MIND (THOUGHTS):

....
....
....

WHAT I NEED FOR MY EMOTIONS (FEELINGS):

....
....
....

WHAT I NEED FOR MY SOUL (DESIRES/DREAMS):

....
....
....

WHAT I NEED FOR MY BODY:

....
....
....

MOVEMENT:

....
....
....

WATER:
GOAL: 1/2 YOUR BODYWEIGHT IN OUNCES

SLEEP:
QUALITY: ☆ ☆ ☆ ☆ ☆ HOURS:.........

NOTES AND REFLECTIONS: ≪

....
....
....
....
....
....
....
....
....
....
....
....
....
....
....
....
....
....
....
....
....
....
....
....
....
....
....
....
....

>> DATE: ....

☐ WRITE THE WORD:

....
....
....
....
....

☐ SOAK IN THE WORD:
SIT. INHALE. EXHALE. MEDITATE ON THIS VERSE FOR 2-3 MINUTES.

☐ WRING IT OUT:
HOW CAN I APPLY THIS VERSE TODAY?

....
....

TODAY I AM GRATEFUL FOR:

☐ 1
....

☐ 2
....

☐ 3
....

TOP 3 THINGS TO DO TODAY:
AS YOU WRITE, VISUALIZE YOURSELF DOING THEM AND THE OUTCOME YOU HOPE FOR.

☐ 1 ....
☐ 2 ....
☐ 3 ....

WHAT I NEED FOR MY MIND (THOUGHTS):

....
....
....

WHAT I NEED FOR MY EMOTIONS (FEELINGS):

....
....
....

WHAT I NEED FOR MY SOUL (DESIRES/DREAMS):

....
....
....

WHAT I NEED FOR MY BODY:

....
....
....

MOVEMENT:

....
....
....

WATER:
GOAL: 1/2 YOUR BODYWEIGHT IN OUNCES

SLEEP:
QUALITY: ☆ ☆ ☆ ☆ ☆ HOURS: ....

NOTES AND REFLECTIONS: «

....
....
....
....
....
....
....
....
....
....
....
....
....
....
....
....
....
....
....
....
....
....
....
....
....
....
....

≫ DATE: ....

☐ WRITE THE WORD:

....
....
....
....
....

☐ SOAK IN THE WORD:
SIT. INHALE. EXHALE. MEDITATE ON THIS VERSE FOR 2-3 MINUTES.

☐ WRING IT OUT:
HOW CAN I APPLY THIS VERSE TODAY?

....
....

TODAY I AM GRATEFUL FOR:

1 ....

2 ....

3 ....

TOP 3 THINGS TO DO TODAY:
AS YOU WRITE, VISUALIZE YOURSELF DOING THEM AND THE OUTCOME YOU HOPE FOR.

1 ....

2 ....

3 ....

WHAT I NEED FOR MY MIND (THOUGHTS):

....

....

....

WHAT I NEED FOR MY EMOTIONS (FEELINGS):

....

....

....

WHAT I NEED FOR MY SOUL (DESIRES/DREAMS):

....

....

....

WHAT I NEED FOR MY BODY:

....

....

....

MOVEMENT:

....

....

....

WATER:
GOAL: 1/2 YOUR BODYWEIGHT IN OUNCES

SLEEP:
QUALITY: ☆ ☆ ☆ ☆ ☆ HOURS: ....

NOTES AND REFLECTIONS: ⟨⟨

....

....

....

....

....

....

....

....

....

....

....

....

....

....

....

....

....

....

....

....

....

....

....

....

....

....

≫ DATE: ....

☐ **WRITE THE WORD:**

....

....

....

....

....

☐ **SOAK IN THE WORD:**
SIT. INHALE. EXHALE. MEDITATE ON THIS VERSE FOR 2-3 MINUTES.

☐ **WRING IT OUT:**
HOW CAN I APPLY THIS VERSE TODAY?

....

....

TODAY I AM GRATEFUL FOR:

1
....

2
....

3
....

TOP 3 THINGS TO DO TODAY:
AS YOU WRITE, VISUALIZE YOURSELF DOING THEM AND THE OUTCOME YOU HOPE FOR.

1
....

2
....

3
....

WHAT I NEED FOR MY MIND (THOUGHTS):

....

....

....

WHAT I NEED FOR MY EMOTIONS (FEELINGS):

....

....

....

WHAT I NEED FOR MY SOUL (DESIRES/DREAMS):

....

....

....

WHAT I NEED FOR MY BODY:

....

....

....

MOVEMENT:

....

....

....

WATER:
GOAL: 1/2 YOUR BODYWEIGHT IN OUNCES

SLEEP:
QUALITY: ☆ ☆ ☆ ☆ ☆ HOURS:.........

NOTES AND REFLECTIONS:

....

....

....

....

....

....

....

....

....

....

....

....

....

....

....

....

....

....

....

....

....

....

....

....

....

....

....

....

>>> DATE:

☐ **WRITE THE WORD:**

....

....

....

....

....

☐ **SOAK IN THE WORD:**
SIT. INHALE. EXHALE. MEDITATE ON THIS VERSE FOR 2-3 MINUTES.

☐ **WRING IT OUT:**
HOW CAN I APPLY THIS VERSE TODAY?

....

....

TODAY I AM GRATEFUL FOR:

1 ....

....

2 ....

....

3 ....

....

TOP 3 THINGS TO DO TODAY:
AS YOU WRITE, VISUALIZE YOURSELF DOING THEM AND THE OUTCOME YOU HOPE FOR.

1 ....

2 ....

3 ....

WHAT I NEED FOR MY MIND (THOUGHTS):

....

....

....

WHAT I NEED FOR MY EMOTIONS (FEELINGS):

....

....

....

WHAT I NEED FOR MY SOUL (DESIRES/DREAMS):

....

....

....

WHAT I NEED FOR MY BODY:

....

....

....

MOVEMENT:

....

....

....

WATER:
GOAL: 1/2 YOUR BODYWEIGHT IN OUNCES

SLEEP:
QUALITY: ☆ ☆ ☆ ☆ ☆ HOURS:..........

NOTES AND REFLECTIONS:

....

....

....

....

....

....

....

....

....

....

....

....

....

....

....

....

....

....

....

....

....

....

....

....

....

....

....

....

≫ DATE: ....

☐ **WRITE THE WORD:**

....

....

....

....

....

☐ **SOAK IN THE WORD:**
SIT. INHALE. EXHALE. MEDITATE ON THIS VERSE FOR 2-3 MINUTES.

☐ **WRING IT OUT:**
HOW CAN I APPLY THIS VERSE TODAY?

....

....

TODAY I AM GRATEFUL FOR:

1 ....

....

2 ....

....

3 ....

....

TOP 3 THINGS TO DO TODAY:
AS YOU WRITE, VISUALIZE YOURSELF DOING THEM AND THE OUTCOME YOU HOPE FOR.

1 ....

2 ....

3 ....

WHAT I NEED FOR MY MIND (THOUGHTS):

....

....

....

WHAT I NEED FOR MY EMOTIONS (FEELINGS):

....

....

....

WHAT I NEED FOR MY SOUL (DESIRES/DREAMS):

....

....

WHAT I NEED FOR MY BODY:

....

....

....

MOVEMENT:

....

....

....

WATER:
GOAL: 1/2 YOUR BODYWEIGHT IN OUNCES

SLEEP:
QUALITY: ☆ ☆ ☆ ☆ ☆ HOURS:.........

NOTES AND REFLECTIONS:

≪

....

....

....

....

....

....

....

....

....

....

....

....

....

....

....

....

....

....

....

....

....

....

....

....

....

≫ DATE: ....

☐ WRITE THE WORD:

....

....

....

....

....

☐ SOAK IN THE WORD:

SIT. INHALE. EXHALE. MEDITATE ON THIS VERSE FOR 2-3 MINUTES.

☐ WRING IT OUT:

HOW CAN I APPLY THIS VERSE TODAY?

....

....

TODAY I AM GRATEFUL FOR:

1 ....

....

2 ....

....

3 ....

....

TOP 3 THINGS TO DO TODAY:

AS YOU WRITE, VISUALIZE YOURSELF DOING THEM AND THE OUTCOME YOU HOPE FOR.

1 ....

2 ....

3 ....

WHAT I NEED FOR MY MIND (THOUGHTS):

....

....

....

WHAT I NEED FOR MY EMOTIONS (FEELINGS):

....

....

....

WHAT I NEED FOR MY SOUL (DESIRES/DREAMS):

....

....

....

WHAT I NEED FOR MY BODY:

....

....

....

MOVEMENT:

....

....

....

WATER:

GOAL: 1/2 YOUR BODYWEIGHT IN OUNCES

SLEEP:
QUALITY: ☆ ☆ ☆ ☆ ☆ HOURS: ....

NOTES AND REFLECTIONS:

....

....

....

....

....

....

....

....

....

....

....

....

....

....

....

....

....

....

....

....

....

....

....

....

....

....

....

≫ DATE: ....

☐ WRITE THE WORD:

....

....

....

....

....

☐ SOAK IN THE WORD:
SIT. INHALE. EXHALE. MEDITATE ON THIS VERSE FOR 2-3 MINUTES.

☐ WRING IT OUT:
HOW CAN I APPLY THIS VERSE TODAY?

....

....

TODAY I AM GRATEFUL FOR:

1 ....

....

2 ....

....

3 ....

....

TOP 3 THINGS TO DO TODAY:
AS YOU WRITE, VISUALIZE YOURSELF DOING THEM AND THE OUTCOME YOU HOPE FOR.

1 ....

2 ....

3 ....

WHAT I NEED FOR MY MIND (THOUGHTS):

....
....
....

WHAT I NEED FOR MY EMOTIONS (FEELINGS):

....
....
....

WHAT I NEED FOR MY SOUL (DESIRES/DREAMS):

....
....
....

WHAT I NEED FOR MY BODY:

....
....
....

MOVEMENT:

....
....
....

WATER:
GOAL: 1/2 YOUR BODYWEIGHT IN OUNCES

SLEEP:
QUALITY: ☆ ☆ ☆ ☆ ☆ HOURS:.........

NOTES AND REFLECTIONS:

....
....
....
....
....
....
....
....
....
....
....
....
....
....
....
....
....
....
....
....
....
....
....
....
....
....

>> DATE:

☐ WRITE THE WORD:

....
....
....
....
....

☐ SOAK IN THE WORD:

SIT. INHALE. EXHALE. MEDITATE ON THIS VERSE FOR 2-3 MINUTES.

☐ WRING IT OUT:

HOW CAN I APPLY THIS VERSE TODAY?

....
....

TODAY I AM GRATEFUL FOR:

1 ....
....

2 ....
....

3 ....
....

TOP 3 THINGS TO DO TODAY:

AS YOU WRITE, VISUALIZE YOURSELF DOING THEM AND THE OUTCOME YOU HOPE FOR.

1 ....

2 ....

3 ....

WHAT I NEED FOR MY MIND (THOUGHTS):

....

....

....

WHAT I NEED FOR MY EMOTIONS (FEELINGS):

....

....

....

WHAT I NEED FOR MY SOUL (DESIRES/DREAMS):

....

....

....

WHAT I NEED FOR MY BODY:

....

....

....

MOVEMENT:

....

....

....

WATER:
GOAL: 1/2 YOUR BODYWEIGHT IN OUNCES

SLEEP:
QUALITY: ☆ ☆ ☆ ☆ ☆ HOURS:..........

NOTES AND REFLECTIONS: ＜＜

....

....

....

....

....

....

....

....

....

....

....

....

....

....

....

....

....

....

....

....

....

....

....

....

....

≫ DATE: ....

☐ **WRITE THE WORD:**

....

....

....

....

....

☐ **SOAK IN THE WORD:**

SIT. INHALE. EXHALE. MEDITATE ON THIS VERSE FOR 2-3 MINUTES.

☐ **WRING IT OUT:**

HOW CAN I APPLY THIS VERSE TODAY?

....

....

TODAY I AM GRATEFUL FOR:

1 ....

....

2 ....

....

3 ....

....

TOP 3 THINGS TO DO TODAY:

AS YOU WRITE, VISUALIZE YOURSELF DOING THEM AND THE OUTCOME YOU HOPE FOR.

1 ....

2 ....

3 ....

WHAT I NEED FOR MY MIND (THOUGHTS):

....

....

....

WHAT I NEED FOR MY EMOTIONS (FEELINGS):

....

....

....

WHAT I NEED FOR MY SOUL (DESIRES/DREAMS):

....

....

....

WHAT I NEED FOR MY BODY:

....

....

....

MOVEMENT:

....

....

....

WATER:
GOAL: 1/2 YOUR BODYWEIGHT IN OUNCES

SLEEP:
QUALITY: ☆ ☆ ☆ ☆ ☆   HOURS: ....

NOTES AND REFLECTIONS: 《

....

....

....

....

....

....

....

....

....

....

....

....

....

....

....

....

....

....

....

....

....

....

....

....

⟫ DATE: ....

☐ WRITE THE WORD:

....
....
....
....
....

☐ SOAK IN THE WORD:

SIT. INHALE. EXHALE. MEDITATE ON THIS VERSE FOR 2-3 MINUTES.

☐ WRING IT OUT:

HOW CAN I APPLY THIS VERSE TODAY?

....
....

TODAY I AM GRATEFUL FOR:

1 ....
2 ....
3 ....

TOP 3 THINGS TO DO TODAY:

AS YOU WRITE, VISUALIZE YOURSELF DOING THEM AND THE OUTCOME YOU HOPE FOR.

1 ....
2 ....
3 ....

WHAT I NEED FOR MY MIND (THOUGHTS):

....
....
....

WHAT I NEED FOR MY EMOTIONS (FEELINGS):

....
....
....

WHAT I NEED FOR MY SOUL (DESIRES/DREAMS):

....
....
....

WHAT I NEED FOR MY BODY:

....
....
....

MOVEMENT:

....
....
....

WATER:
GOAL: 1/2 YOUR BODYWEIGHT IN OUNCES

SLEEP:
QUALITY: ☆ ☆ ☆ ☆ ☆ HOURS:.........

NOTES AND REFLECTIONS: 《《

....
....
....
....
....
....
....
....
....
....
....
....
....
....
....
....
....
....
....
....
....
....
....
....
....
....

≫ DATE: ....

☐ WRITE THE WORD:

....
....
....
....
....

☐ SOAK IN THE WORD:
SIT. INHALE. EXHALE. MEDITATE ON THIS VERSE FOR 2-3 MINUTES.

☐ WRING IT OUT:
HOW CAN I APPLY THIS VERSE TODAY?

....
....

TODAY I AM GRATEFUL FOR:

1
....

2
....

3
....

TOP 3 THINGS TO DO TODAY:
AS YOU WRITE, VISUALIZE YOURSELF DOING THEM AND THE OUTCOME YOU HOPE FOR.

1
....
2
....
3
....

WHAT I NEED FOR MY MIND (THOUGHTS):

....

....

....

WHAT I NEED FOR MY EMOTIONS (FEELINGS):

....

....

....

WHAT I NEED FOR MY SOUL (DESIRES/DREAMS):

....

....

....

WHAT I NEED FOR MY BODY:

....

....

....

MOVEMENT:

....

....

....

WATER:
GOAL: 1/2 YOUR BODYWEIGHT IN OUNCES

SLEEP:
QUALITY: ☆ ☆ ☆ ☆ ☆ HOURS:.........

NOTES AND REFLECTIONS:

....

....

....

....

....

....

....

....

....

....

....

....

....

....

....

....

....

....

....

....

....

....

....

....

....

....

≫ DATE: ....

☐ **WRITE THE WORD:**

....

....

....

....

....

☐ **SOAK IN THE WORD:**
SIT. INHALE. EXHALE. MEDITATE ON THIS VERSE FOR 2-3 MINUTES.

☐ **WRING IT OUT:**
HOW CAN I APPLY THIS VERSE TODAY?

....

....

TODAY I AM GRATEFUL FOR:

1 ....

2 ....

3 ....

....

TOP 3 THINGS TO DO TODAY:
AS YOU WRITE, VISUALIZE YOURSELF DOING THEM AND THE OUTCOME YOU HOPE FOR.

1 ....

2 ....

3 ....

WHAT I NEED FOR MY MIND (THOUGHTS):

....

....

....

WHAT I NEED FOR MY EMOTIONS (FEELINGS):

....

....

....

WHAT I NEED FOR MY SOUL (DESIRES/DREAMS):

....

....

....

WHAT I NEED FOR MY BODY:

....

....

....

MOVEMENT:

....

....

....

WATER:
GOAL: 1/2 YOUR BODYWEIGHT IN OUNCES

SLEEP:
QUALITY: ☆ ☆ ☆ ☆ ☆ HOURS: ....

NOTES AND REFLECTIONS: 《

....

....

....

....

....

....

....

....

....

....

....

....

....

....

....

....

....

....

....

....

....

....

....

....

....

≫ DATE: ....

☐ WRITE THE WORD:

....
....
....
....
....

☐ SOAK IN THE WORD:
   SIT. INHALE. EXHALE. MEDITATE ON THIS VERSE FOR 2-3 MINUTES.

☐ WRING IT OUT:
   HOW CAN I APPLY THIS VERSE TODAY?

....
....

TODAY I AM GRATEFUL FOR:

1 ....
....

2 ....
....

3 ....
....

TOP 3 THINGS TO DO TODAY:
AS YOU WRITE, VISUALIZE YOURSELF DOING THEM AND THE OUTCOME YOU HOPE FOR.

1 ....

2 ....

3 ....

WHAT I NEED FOR MY MIND (THOUGHTS):

....

....

....

WHAT I NEED FOR MY EMOTIONS (FEELINGS):

....

....

....

WHAT I NEED FOR MY SOUL (DESIRES/DREAMS):

....

....

....

WHAT I NEED FOR MY BODY:

....

....

....

MOVEMENT:

....

....

....

WATER:
GOAL: 1/2 YOUR BODYWEIGHT IN OUNCES

SLEEP:
QUALITY: ☆ ☆ ☆ ☆ ☆ HOURS:.........

NOTES AND REFLECTIONS: «

....

....

....

....

....

....

....

....

....

....

....

....

....

....

....

....

....

....

....

....

....

....

....

....

....

....

》》 DATE: ....

☐ WRITE THE WORD:

....

....

....

....

....

☐ SOAK IN THE WORD:
SIT. INHALE. EXHALE. MEDITATE ON THIS VERSE FOR 2-3 MINUTES.

☐ WRING IT OUT:
HOW CAN I APPLY THIS VERSE TODAY?

....

....

TODAY I AM GRATEFUL FOR:

1 ....

2 ....

3 ....

TOP 3 THINGS TO DO TODAY:
AS YOU WRITE, VISUALIZE YOURSELF DOING THEM AND THE OUTCOME YOU HOPE FOR.

1 ....

2 ....

3 ....

WHAT I NEED FOR MY MIND (THOUGHTS):

....
....
....

WHAT I NEED FOR MY EMOTIONS (FEELINGS):

....
....
....

WHAT I NEED FOR MY SOUL (DESIRES/DREAMS):

....
....
....

WHAT I NEED FOR MY BODY:

....
....
....

MOVEMENT:

....
....
....

WATER:
GOAL: 1/2 YOUR BODYWEIGHT IN OUNCES

SLEEP:
QUALITY: ☆ ☆ ☆ ☆ ☆ HOURS:.........

NOTES AND REFLECTIONS:

....
....
....
....
....
....
....
....
....
....
....
....
....
....
....
....
....
....
....
....
....
....
....
....
....
....
....

≫ DATE: ....

☐ WRITE THE WORD:

....
....
....
....
....

☐ SOAK IN THE WORD:
SIT. INHALE. EXHALE. MEDITATE ON THIS VERSE FOR 2-3 MINUTES.

☐ WRING IT OUT:
HOW CAN I APPLY THIS VERSE TODAY?

....
....

TODAY I AM GRATEFUL FOR:

1
....

2
....

3
....

TOP 3 THINGS TO DO TODAY:
AS YOU WRITE, VISUALIZE YOURSELF DOING THEM AND THE OUTCOME YOU HOPE FOR.

1 ....
2 ....
3 ....

WHAT I NEED FOR MY MIND (THOUGHTS):

....

....

WHAT I NEED FOR MY EMOTIONS (FEELINGS):

....

....

....

WHAT I NEED FOR MY SOUL (DESIRES/DREAMS):

....

....

....

WHAT I NEED FOR MY BODY:

....

....

....

MOVEMENT:

....

....

....

WATER:
GOAL: 1/2 YOUR BODYWEIGHT IN OUNCES

SLEEP:
QUALITY: ☆ ☆ ☆ ☆ ☆ HOURS: ....

NOTES AND REFLECTIONS:

....

....

....

....

....

....

....

....

....

....

....

....

....

....

....

....

....

....

....

....

....

....

....

....

....

≫ DATE: ....

☐ **WRITE THE WORD:**

....

....

....

....

....

☐ **SOAK IN THE WORD:**
SIT. INHALE. EXHALE. MEDITATE ON THIS VERSE FOR 2-3 MINUTES.

☐ **WRING IT OUT:**
HOW CAN I APPLY THIS VERSE TODAY?

....

....

TODAY I AM GRATEFUL FOR:

1
....

....

2
....

....

3
....

....

TOP 3 THINGS TO DO TODAY:
AS YOU WRITE, VISUALIZE YOURSELF DOING THEM AND THE OUTCOME YOU HOPE FOR.

1
....

2
....

3
....

WHAT I NEED FOR MY MIND (THOUGHTS):

....

....

....

WHAT I NEED FOR MY EMOTIONS (FEELINGS):

....

....

....

WHAT I NEED FOR MY SOUL (DESIRES/DREAMS):

....

....

....

WHAT I NEED FOR MY BODY:

....

....

....

MOVEMENT:

....

....

....

WATER:
GOAL: 1/2 YOUR BODYWEIGHT IN OUNCES

SLEEP:
QUALITY: ☆ ☆ ☆ ☆ ☆ HOURS: ....

NOTES AND REFLECTIONS:

....

....

....

....

....

....

....

....

....

....

....

....

....

....

....

....

....

....

....

....

....

....

....

....

....

....

....

≫ DATE: ....

☐ **WRITE THE WORD:**

....
....
....
....
....

☐ **SOAK IN THE WORD:**
   SIT. INHALE. EXHALE. MEDITATE ON THIS VERSE FOR 2-3 MINUTES.

☐ **WRING IT OUT:**
   HOW CAN I APPLY THIS VERSE TODAY?

....
....

TODAY I AM GRATEFUL FOR:

1 ....

2 ....

3 ....

TOP 3 THINGS TO DO TODAY:
AS YOU WRITE, VISUALIZE YOURSELF DOING THEM AND THE OUTCOME YOU HOPE FOR.

1 ....

2 ....

3 ....

WHAT I NEED FOR MY MIND (THOUGHTS):

....

....

....

WHAT I NEED FOR MY EMOTIONS (FEELINGS):

....

....

....

WHAT I NEED FOR MY SOUL (DESIRES/DREAMS):

....

....

....

WHAT I NEED FOR MY BODY:

....

....

....

MOVEMENT:

....

....

....

WATER:
GOAL: 1/2 YOUR BODYWEIGHT IN OUNCES

SLEEP:
QUALITY: ☆ ☆ ☆ ☆ ☆ HOURS: ....

NOTES AND REFLECTIONS: ≪

....

....

....

....

....

....

....

....

....

....

....

....

....

....

....

....

....

....

....

....

....

....

....

....

....

....

....

⟫ DATE: ....

☐ WRITE THE WORD:

....
....
....
....
....

☐ SOAK IN THE WORD:
SIT. INHALE. EXHALE. MEDITATE ON THIS VERSE FOR 2-3 MINUTES.

☐ WRING IT OUT:
HOW CAN I APPLY THIS VERSE TODAY?

....
....

TODAY I AM GRATEFUL FOR:
1 ....
....

2 ....
....

3 ....
....

TOP 3 THINGS TO DO TODAY:
AS YOU WRITE, VISUALIZE YOURSELF DOING THEM AND THE OUTCOME YOU HOPE FOR.

1 ....
2 ....
3 ....

WHAT I NEED FOR MY MIND (THOUGHTS):

....

....

....

WHAT I NEED FOR MY EMOTIONS (FEELINGS):

....

....

....

WHAT I NEED FOR MY SOUL (DESIRES/DREAMS):

....

....

....

WHAT I NEED FOR MY BODY:

....

....

....

MOVEMENT:

....

....

....

WATER:
GOAL: 1/2 YOUR BODYWEIGHT IN OUNCES

SLEEP:
QUALITY: ☆☆☆☆☆ HOURS:.........

NOTES AND REFLECTIONS: 《《

....

....

....

....

....

....

....

....

....

....

....

....

....

....

....

....

....

....

....

....

....

....

....

....

....

....

≫ DATE: ....

☐ **WRITE THE WORD:**

....
....
....
....
....

☐ **SOAK IN THE WORD:**
   SIT. INHALE. EXHALE. MEDITATE ON THIS VERSE FOR 2-3 MINUTES.

☐ **WRING IT OUT:**
   HOW CAN I APPLY THIS VERSE TODAY?

....
....

TODAY I AM GRATEFUL FOR:

1 ....

2 ....

3 ....

TOP 3 THINGS TO DO TODAY:
AS YOU WRITE, VISUALIZE YOURSELF DOING THEM AND THE OUTCOME YOU HOPE FOR.

1 ....
2 ....
3 ....

WHAT I NEED FOR MY MIND (THOUGHTS):

....

....

....

WHAT I NEED FOR MY EMOTIONS (FEELINGS):

....

....

....

WHAT I NEED FOR MY SOUL (DESIRES/DREAMS):

....

....

....

WHAT I NEED FOR MY BODY:

....

....

....

MOVEMENT:

....

....

....

WATER:
GOAL: 1/2 YOUR BODYWEIGHT IN OUNCES

SLEEP:
QUALITY: ☆ ☆ ☆ ☆ ☆ HOURS:.........

NOTES AND REFLECTIONS: ≪

....

....

....

....

....

....

....

....

....

....

....

....

....

....

....

....

....

....

....

....

....

....

....

....

....

....

»» DATE: ....

☐ WRITE THE WORD:

....

....

....

....

....

☐ SOAK IN THE WORD:
SIT. INHALE. EXHALE. MEDITATE ON THIS VERSE FOR 2-3 MINUTES.

☐ WRING IT OUT:
HOW CAN I APPLY THIS VERSE TODAY?

....

....

TODAY I AM GRATEFUL FOR:

1
....

2
....

3
....

TOP 3 THINGS TO DO TODAY:
AS YOU WRITE, VISUALIZE YOURSELF DOING THEM AND THE OUTCOME YOU HOPE FOR.

1
....

2
....

3
....

WHAT I NEED FOR MY MIND (THOUGHTS):

....

....

....

WHAT I NEED FOR MY EMOTIONS (FEELINGS):

....

....

....

WHAT I NEED FOR MY SOUL (DESIRES/DREAMS):

....

....

....

WHAT I NEED FOR MY BODY:

....

....

....

MOVEMENT:

....

....

....

WATER:
GOAL: 1/2 YOUR BODYWEIGHT IN OUNCES

SLEEP:
QUALITY: ☆ ☆ ☆ ☆ ☆ HOURS: ....

NOTES AND REFLECTIONS: 《

....

....

....

....

....

....

....

....

....

....

....

....

....

....

....

....

....

....

....

....

....

....

....

....

....

⟫ DATE: ....

☐ **WRITE THE WORD:**

....
....
....
....
....

☐ **SOAK IN THE WORD:**
SIT. INHALE. EXHALE. MEDITATE ON THIS VERSE FOR 2-3 MINUTES.

☐ **WRING IT OUT:**
HOW CAN I APPLY THIS VERSE TODAY?

....
....

TODAY I AM GRATEFUL FOR:

1
....

2
....

3
....

TOP 3 THINGS TO DO TODAY:
AS YOU WRITE, VISUALIZE YOURSELF DOING THEM AND THE OUTCOME YOU HOPE FOR.

1 ....
2 ....
3 ....

WHAT I NEED FOR MY MIND (THOUGHTS):

....

....

....

WHAT I NEED FOR MY EMOTIONS (FEELINGS):

....

....

....

WHAT I NEED FOR MY SOUL (DESIRES/DREAMS):

....

....

....

WHAT I NEED FOR MY BODY:

....

....

....

MOVEMENT:

....

....

....

WATER:
GOAL: 1/2 YOUR BODYWEIGHT IN OUNCES

SLEEP:
QUALITY: ☆ ☆ ☆ ☆ ☆ HOURS:..........

NOTES AND REFLECTIONS: ≪

....

....

....

....

....

....

....

....

....

....

....

....

....

....

....

....

....

....

....

....

....

....

....

....

....

....

....

≫ DATE: ....

☐ WRITE THE WORD:

....

....

....

....

....

☐ SOAK IN THE WORD:
SIT. INHALE. EXHALE. MEDITATE ON THIS VERSE FOR 2-3 MINUTES.

☐ WRING IT OUT:
HOW CAN I APPLY THIS VERSE TODAY?

....

....

TODAY I AM GRATEFUL FOR:

1
....

2
....

3
....

TOP 3 THINGS TO DO TODAY:
AS YOU WRITE, VISUALIZE YOURSELF DOING THEM AND THE OUTCOME YOU HOPE FOR.

1
....

2
....

3
....

WHAT I NEED FOR MY MIND (THOUGHTS):

....
....
....

WHAT I NEED FOR MY EMOTIONS (FEELINGS):

....
....
....

WHAT I NEED FOR MY SOUL (DESIRES/DREAMS):

....
....
....

WHAT I NEED FOR MY BODY:

....
....
....

MOVEMENT:

....
....
....

WATER:
GOAL: 1/2 YOUR BODYWEIGHT IN OUNCES

SLEEP:
QUALITY: ☆ ☆ ☆ ☆ ☆ HOURS:.........

NOTES AND REFLECTIONS: ≪

....
....
....
....
....
....
....
....
....
....
....
....
....
....
....
....
....
....
....
....
....
....
....
....

≫ DATE: ....

☐ WRITE THE WORD:

....
....
....
....
....

☐ SOAK IN THE WORD:

SIT. INHALE. EXHALE. MEDITATE ON THIS VERSE FOR 2-3 MINUTES.

☐ WRING IT OUT:

HOW CAN I APPLY THIS VERSE TODAY?

....
....

TODAY I AM GRATEFUL FOR:

1 ....

2 ....

3 ....

TOP 3 THINGS TO DO TODAY:

AS YOU WRITE, VISUALIZE YOURSELF DOING THEM AND THE OUTCOME YOU HOPE FOR.

1 ....

2 ....

3 ....

WHAT I NEED FOR MY MIND (THOUGHTS):

....

....

....

WHAT I NEED FOR MY EMOTIONS (FEELINGS):

....

....

....

WHAT I NEED FOR MY SOUL (DESIRES/DREAMS):

....

....

....

WHAT I NEED FOR MY BODY:

....

....

....

MOVEMENT:

....

....

....

WATER:
GOAL: 1/2 YOUR BODYWEIGHT IN OUNCES

SLEEP:
QUALITY: ☆ ☆ ☆ ☆ ☆ HOURS:.........

NOTES AND REFLECTIONS: ⟪

....

....

....

....

....

....

....

....

....

....

....

....

....

....

....

....

....

....

....

....

....

....

....

....

≫ DATE: ....

☐ WRITE THE WORD:

....
....
....
....
....

☐ SOAK IN THE WORD:
SIT. INHALE. EXHALE. MEDITATE ON THIS VERSE FOR 2-3 MINUTES.

☐ WRING IT OUT:
HOW CAN I APPLY THIS VERSE TODAY?

....
....

TODAY I AM GRATEFUL FOR:

1 ....

2 ....

3 ....

TOP 3 THINGS TO DO TODAY:
AS YOU WRITE, VISUALIZE YOURSELF DOING THEM AND THE OUTCOME YOU HOPE FOR.

1 ....

2 ....

3 ....

WHAT I NEED FOR MY MIND (THOUGHTS):

....

....

WHAT I NEED FOR MY EMOTIONS (FEELINGS):

....

....

....

WHAT I NEED FOR MY SOUL (DESIRES/DREAMS):

....

....

....

WHAT I NEED FOR MY BODY:

....

....

....

MOVEMENT:

....

....

....

WATER:
GOAL: 1/2 YOUR BODYWEIGHT IN OUNCES

SLEEP:
QUALITY: ☆☆☆☆☆ HOURS: ....

NOTES AND REFLECTIONS:

....

....

....

....

....

....

....

....

....

....

....

....

....

....

....

....

....

....

....

....

....

....

....

....

....

....

≫ DATE: ....

☐ WRITE THE WORD:

....

....

....

....

....

☐ SOAK IN THE WORD:
SIT. INHALE. EXHALE. MEDITATE ON THIS VERSE FOR 2-3 MINUTES.

☐ WRING IT OUT:
HOW CAN I APPLY THIS VERSE TODAY?

....

....

TODAY I AM GRATEFUL FOR:

1
....

2
....

3
....

TOP 3 THINGS TO DO TODAY:
AS YOU WRITE, VISUALIZE YOURSELF DOING THEM AND THE OUTCOME YOU HOPE FOR.

1
....

2
....

3
....

WHAT I NEED FOR MY MIND (THOUGHTS):

....

....

....

WHAT I NEED FOR MY EMOTIONS (FEELINGS):

....

....

....

WHAT I NEED FOR MY SOUL (DESIRES/DREAMS):

....

....

....

WHAT I NEED FOR MY BODY:

....

....

....

MOVEMENT:

....

....

....

WATER:
GOAL: 1/2 YOUR BODYWEIGHT IN OUNCES

SLEEP:
QUALITY: ☆ ☆ ☆ ☆ ☆ HOURS:.........

NOTES AND REFLECTIONS: 《《

....

....

....

....

....

....

....

....

....

....

....

....

....

....

....

....

....

....

....

....

....

....

....

....

....

....

....

....

....

≫ DATE: ....

☐ **WRITE THE WORD:**

....

....

....

....

....

☐ **SOAK IN THE WORD:**
   SIT. INHALE. EXHALE. MEDITATE ON THIS VERSE FOR 2-3 MINUTES.

☐ **WRING IT OUT:**
   HOW CAN I APPLY THIS VERSE TODAY?

....

....

TODAY I AM GRATEFUL FOR:

1 ....

2 ....

3 ....

TOP 3 THINGS TO DO TODAY:
AS YOU WRITE, VISUALIZE YOURSELF DOING THEM AND THE OUTCOME YOU HOPE FOR.

1 ....

2 ....

3 ....

WHAT I NEED FOR MY MIND (THOUGHTS):

....
....
....

WHAT I NEED FOR MY EMOTIONS (FEELINGS):

....
....
....

WHAT I NEED FOR MY SOUL (DESIRES/DREAMS):

....
....
....

WHAT I NEED FOR MY BODY:

....
....
....

MOVEMENT:

....
....
....

WATER:
GOAL: 1/2 YOUR BODYWEIGHT IN OUNCES

SLEEP:
QUALITY: ☆ ☆ ☆ ☆ ☆ HOURS:.........

NOTES AND REFLECTIONS: ‹‹‹

....
....
....
....
....
....
....
....
....
....
....
....
....
....
....
....
....
....
....
....
....
....
....
....
....
....

≫ DATE: ....

☐ WRITE THE WORD:

....

....

....

....

....

☐ SOAK IN THE WORD:
SIT. INHALE. EXHALE. MEDITATE ON THIS VERSE FOR 2-3 MINUTES.

☐ WRING IT OUT:
HOW CAN I APPLY THIS VERSE TODAY?

....

....

TODAY I AM GRATEFUL FOR:

1 ....

2 ....

3 ....

TOP 3 THINGS TO DO TODAY:
AS YOU WRITE, VISUALIZE YOURSELF DOING THEM AND THE OUTCOME YOU HOPE FOR.

1 ....

2 ....

3 ....

WHAT I NEED FOR MY MIND (THOUGHTS):

....
....
....

WHAT I NEED FOR MY EMOTIONS (FEELINGS):

....
....
....

WHAT I NEED FOR MY SOUL (DESIRES/DREAMS):

....
....
....

WHAT I NEED FOR MY BODY:

....
....
....

MOVEMENT:

....
....
....

WATER:
GOAL: 1/2 YOUR BODYWEIGHT IN OUNCES

SLEEP:
QUALITY: ☆ ☆ ☆ ☆ ☆ HOURS:.........

NOTES AND REFLECTIONS: 《《

....
....
....
....
....
....
....
....
....
....
....
....
....
....
....
....
....
....
....
....
....
....
....
....
....

≫ DATE: ....

☐ WRITE THE WORD:

....

....

....

....

....

☐ SOAK IN THE WORD:
SIT. INHALE. EXHALE. MEDITATE ON THIS VERSE FOR 2-3 MINUTES.

☐ WRING IT OUT:
HOW CAN I APPLY THIS VERSE TODAY?

....

....

TODAY I AM GRATEFUL FOR:

1 ....

2 ....

3 ....

TOP 3 THINGS TO DO TODAY:
AS YOU WRITE, VISUALIZE YOURSELF DOING THEM AND THE OUTCOME YOU HOPE FOR.

1 ....

2 ....

3 ....

WHAT I NEED FOR MY MIND (THOUGHTS):

....

....

....

WHAT I NEED FOR MY EMOTIONS (FEELINGS):

....

....

....

WHAT I NEED FOR MY SOUL (DESIRES/DREAMS):

....

....

....

WHAT I NEED FOR MY BODY:

....

....

....

MOVEMENT:

....

....

....

WATER:
GOAL: 1/2 YOUR BODYWEIGHT IN OUNCES

SLEEP:
QUALITY: ☆☆☆☆☆ HOURS:.........

NOTES AND REFLECTIONS:

....

....

....

....

....

....

....

....

....

....

....

....

....

....

....

....

....

....

....

....

....

....

....

....

....

....

....

≫ DATE: ....

☐ **WRITE THE WORD:**

....

....

....

....

....

☐ **SOAK IN THE WORD:**
SIT. INHALE. EXHALE. MEDITATE ON THIS VERSE FOR 2-3 MINUTES.

☐ **WRING IT OUT:**
HOW CAN I APPLY THIS VERSE TODAY?

....

....

TODAY I AM GRATEFUL FOR:

1 ....

2 ....

3 ....

TOP 3 THINGS TO DO TODAY:
AS YOU WRITE, VISUALIZE YOURSELF DOING THEM AND THE OUTCOME YOU HOPE FOR.

1 ....

2 ....

3 ....

WHAT I NEED FOR MY MIND (THOUGHTS):

....

....

....

WHAT I NEED FOR MY EMOTIONS (FEELINGS):

....

....

....

WHAT I NEED FOR MY SOUL (DESIRES/DREAMS):

....

....

....

WHAT I NEED FOR MY BODY:

....

....

....

MOVEMENT:

....

....

....

WATER:
GOAL: 1/2 YOUR BODYWEIGHT IN OUNCES

SLEEP:
QUALITY: ☆ ☆ ☆ ☆ ☆ HOURS:.........

NOTES AND REFLECTIONS: ⟪

....

....

....

....

....

....

....

....

....

....

....

....

....

....

....

....

....

....

....

....

....

....

....

....

....

≫ DATE: ....

☐ **WRITE THE WORD:**

....
....
....
....
....

☐ **SOAK IN THE WORD:**
SIT. INHALE. EXHALE. MEDITATE ON THIS VERSE FOR 2-3 MINUTES.

☐ **WRING IT OUT:**
HOW CAN I APPLY THIS VERSE TODAY?

....
....

TODAY I AM GRATEFUL FOR:

1 ....
....

2 ....
....

3 ....
....

TOP 3 THINGS TO DO TODAY:
AS YOU WRITE, VISUALIZE YOURSELF DOING THEM AND THE OUTCOME YOU HOPE FOR.

1 ....

2 ....

3 ....

WHAT I NEED FOR MY MIND (THOUGHTS):

....
....
....

WHAT I NEED FOR MY EMOTIONS (FEELINGS):

....
....
....

WHAT I NEED FOR MY SOUL (DESIRES/DREAMS):

....
....
....

WHAT I NEED FOR MY BODY:

....
....
....

MOVEMENT:

....
....
....

WATER:
GOAL: 1/2 YOUR BODYWEIGHT IN OUNCES

SLEEP:
QUALITY: ☆ ☆ ☆ ☆ ☆ HOURS: ....

NOTES AND REFLECTIONS: 《《

....
....
....
....
....
....
....
....
....
....
....
....
....
....
....
....
....
....
....
....
....
....
....
....
....
....
....

≫ DATE: ....

☐ **WRITE THE WORD:**

....
....
....
....
....

☐ **SOAK IN THE WORD:**
SIT. INHALE. EXHALE. MEDITATE ON THIS VERSE FOR 2-3 MINUTES.

☐ **WRING IT OUT:**
HOW CAN I APPLY THIS VERSE TODAY?

....
....

TODAY I AM GRATEFUL FOR:

1 ....

2 ....

3 ....

TOP 3 THINGS TO DO TODAY:
AS YOU WRITE, VISUALIZE YOURSELF DOING THEM AND THE OUTCOME YOU HOPE FOR.

1 ....

2 ....

3 ....

WHAT I NEED FOR MY MIND (THOUGHTS):

....
....
....

WHAT I NEED FOR MY EMOTIONS (FEELINGS):

....
....
....

WHAT I NEED FOR MY SOUL (DESIRES/DREAMS):

....
....
....

WHAT I NEED FOR MY BODY:

....
....
....

MOVEMENT:

....
....
....

WATER:
GOAL: 1/2 YOUR BODYWEIGHT IN OUNCES

SLEEP:
QUALITY: ☆ ☆ ☆ ☆ ☆ HOURS:.........

NOTES AND REFLECTIONS: ≪

....
....
....
....
....
....
....
....
....
....
....
....
....
....
....
....
....
....
....
....
....
....
....
....
....
....
....

≫ DATE: ....

☐ **WRITE THE WORD:**

....
....
....
....
....

☐ **SOAK IN THE WORD:**
   SIT. INHALE. EXHALE. MEDITATE ON THIS VERSE FOR 2-3 MINUTES.

☐ **WRING IT OUT:**
   HOW CAN I APPLY THIS VERSE TODAY?

....
....

TODAY I AM GRATEFUL FOR:

1 ....

2 ....

3 ....
....

TOP 3 THINGS TO DO TODAY:
AS YOU WRITE, VISUALIZE YOURSELF DOING THEM AND THE OUTCOME YOU HOPE FOR.

1 ....
2 ....
3 ....

WHAT I NEED FOR MY MIND (THOUGHTS):

....

....

....

WHAT I NEED FOR MY EMOTIONS (FEELINGS):

....

....

....

WHAT I NEED FOR MY SOUL (DESIRES/DREAMS):

....

....

....

WHAT I NEED FOR MY BODY:

....

....

....

MOVEMENT:

....

....

....

WATER:
GOAL: 1/2 YOUR BODYWEIGHT IN OUNCES

SLEEP:
QUALITY: ☆ ☆ ☆ ☆ ☆ HOURS: ....

NOTES AND REFLECTIONS: 《

....

....

....

....

....

....

....

....

....

....

....

....

....

....

....

....

....

....

....

....

....

....

....

....

....

....

⟫ DATE: ....

☐ **WRITE THE WORD:**

....
....
....
....
....

☐ **SOAK IN THE WORD:**
   SIT. INHALE. EXHALE. MEDITATE ON THIS VERSE FOR 2-3 MINUTES.

☐ **WRING IT OUT:**
   HOW CAN I APPLY THIS VERSE TODAY?

....
....

TODAY I AM GRATEFUL FOR:

1 ....

2 ....

3 ....

TOP 3 THINGS TO DO TODAY:
AS YOU WRITE, VISUALIZE YOURSELF DOING THEM AND THE OUTCOME YOU HOPE FOR.

1 ....

2 ....

3 ....

WHAT I NEED FOR MY MIND (THOUGHTS):

....

....

....

WHAT I NEED FOR MY EMOTIONS (FEELINGS):

....

....

....

WHAT I NEED FOR MY SOUL (DESIRES/DREAMS):

....

....

....

WHAT I NEED FOR MY BODY:

....

....

....

MOVEMENT:

....

....

....

WATER:
GOAL: 1/2 YOUR BODYWEIGHT IN OUNCES

SLEEP:
QUALITY: ☆ ☆ ☆ ☆ ☆ HOURS:.........

NOTES AND REFLECTIONS:

....

....

....

....

....

....

....

....

....

....

....

....

....

....

....

....

....

....

....

....

....

....

....

....

....

....

≫ DATE: ....

☐ WRITE THE WORD:

....

....

....

....

....

☐ SOAK IN THE WORD:
SIT. INHALE. EXHALE. MEDITATE ON THIS VERSE FOR 2-3 MINUTES.

☐ WRING IT OUT:
HOW CAN I APPLY THIS VERSE TODAY?

....

....

TODAY I AM GRATEFUL FOR:

1
....

2
....

3
....

....

TOP 3 THINGS TO DO TODAY:
AS YOU WRITE, VISUALIZE YOURSELF DOING THEM AND THE OUTCOME YOU HOPE FOR.

1
....

2
....

3
....

WHAT I NEED FOR MY MIND (THOUGHTS):

....

....

....

WHAT I NEED FOR MY EMOTIONS (FEELINGS):

....

....

....

WHAT I NEED FOR MY SOUL (DESIRES/DREAMS):

....

....

....

WHAT I NEED FOR MY BODY:

....

....

....

MOVEMENT:

....

....

....

WATER:
GOAL: 1/2 YOUR BODYWEIGHT IN OUNCES

SLEEP:
QUALITY: ☆ ☆ ☆ ☆ ☆ HOURS: ....

NOTES AND REFLECTIONS:

....

....

....

....

....

....

....

....

....

....

....

....

....

....

....

....

....

....

....

....

....

....

....

....

≫ DATE: ....

☐ WRITE THE WORD:

....

....

....

....

....

☐ SOAK IN THE WORD:

SIT. INHALE. EXHALE. MEDITATE ON THIS VERSE FOR 2-3 MINUTES.

☐ WRING IT OUT:

HOW CAN I APPLY THIS VERSE TODAY?

....

....

TODAY I AM GRATEFUL FOR:

1
....

2
....

3
....

TOP 3 THINGS TO DO TODAY:

AS YOU WRITE, VISUALIZE YOURSELF DOING THEM AND THE OUTCOME YOU HOPE FOR.

1
....

2
....

3
....

WHAT I NEED FOR MY MIND (THOUGHTS):

....
....
....

WHAT I NEED FOR MY EMOTIONS (FEELINGS):

....
....
....

WHAT I NEED FOR MY SOUL (DESIRES/DREAMS):

....
....
....

WHAT I NEED FOR MY BODY:

....
....
....

MOVEMENT:

....
....
....

WATER:
GOAL: 1/2 YOUR BODYWEIGHT IN OUNCES

SLEEP:
QUALITY: ☆ ☆ ☆ ☆ ☆ HOURS:..........

NOTES AND REFLECTIONS:

....
....
....
....
....
....
....
....
....
....
....
....
....
....
....
....
....
....
....
....
....
....
....
....
....
....

CONNECT WITH US

 www.revelationwellness.org

facebook.com/revelationwell

instagram.com/revelationwellness

Made in the USA
Las Vegas, NV
06 January 2024

83985856R00055